KICK START FOR WEIGHT LOSS

3 MASSIVE MISTAKES PROFESSIONAL WOMEN MAKE
THAT KEEP THEM OVERWEIGHT, EXHAUSTED AND STUCK
ON THE DIET TREADMILL

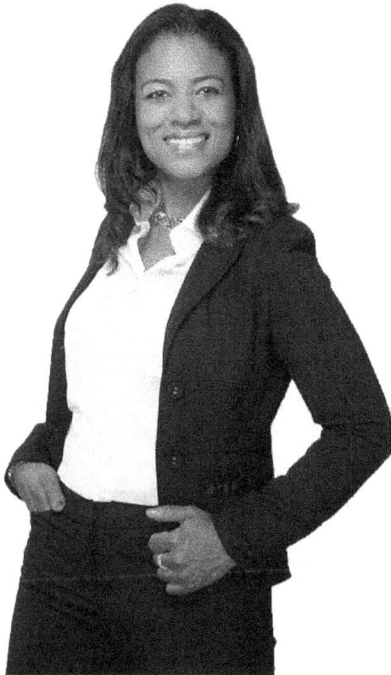

MONIQUE BARTLETT

Praise for Kick Start For Weight Loss

From Mistake #3 to Mistake #1, I was captivated. Kick Start For Weight Loss: 3 Massive Mistakes Professional Women Make That Keep Them Overweight, Exhausted and Stuck On The Diet Treadmill is a real eye opener. Monique provides you with a game plan to create the results you want. ---

Karen E. Grant, Author of The Million Dollar Image, How To Step Into A More Powerful Persona

Monique has really put together one of the most practical books I have come across. The worksheets and exercises in this book are really great. Use them yourself and then share them with your friends and family ---

Dr. Justine Blainey, Owner, Justine Blainey Wellness Centre

Get a clear line of action of what to do to help you reach your weight loss goal. If you need direction, then read this book from beginning to end! ---

Lori Kennedy, Owner, Wow Weight Loss

I have worked with Monique Bartlett and have had the pleasure to experience the passion she has in her business. She has tremendous skills and knowledge. She gently, yet firmly leads women to greater success than they can imagine. ---

Jan Freethy, Owner, Jan Freethy

This book will get you to see more clearly that you can clear away any obstacle that holds you back so you can achieve your weight loss goal. ---

Dina Vieira, President, DV Communications

Monique shows how changing your mindset and habits can be so simple and manageable. If you want to stop being overweight, exhausted and stuck on the diet treadmill, then this book is a must read! ---

Erica Mitchell, Former Client

This book proves that everything is possible with the right mindset. ---

Duanyi Wu, Owner, Duanyi Coaching

You don't have to lose weight to be healthy – you have to be healthy to lose weight and that includes changing certain belief systems. Kick Start For Weight Loss provides valuable tools and information on how to breakthrough old patterns that are holding you back from achieving your weight loss goals.---

Dr. Natasha Turner ND, Best Selling Author of The Hormone Diet

ISBN 978-0-9936421-0-4

Published by 2 The Core Publications

The information contained herein is intended for informational purposes only and should not be relied upon by recipients hereof. Although the information is believed to be correct, its accuracy, correctness or completeness cannot be guaranteed. The author designed the information to represent her opinions about the subjects disclosed. The reader must weigh carefully all aspects of any personal decision before making any changes in their life. The author obtained the information contained through education and experience and speaks from her experience and perspective only.

The author disclaims any liability, loss or risk incurred by any readers who act on the information enclosed. As each individual situation is unique, questions relevant to a specific situation should be addressed to an appropriate professional to ensure their situation has been evaluated carefully and appropriately.

Go to

www.moniquebartlett.com

Discover workshops and programs that can help you achieve your
goals. Don't wait. Go to www.moniquebartlett.com today!

**COMPANIES, ORGANIZATIONS, INSTITUTIONS AND INDUSTRY
PUBLICATIONS:** Discounts are available on bulk purchases of this
book for reselling, educational purposes, subscription incentives,
gifts, sponsorship or fundraising. Special books or book excerpts can
also be created to fit specific needs. For more information please
contact: **info@moniquebartlett.com**

Dedication

This book is dedicated to any professional woman who has consistently struggled with being exhausted and overweight. If you thought that you could never achieve your ideal weight, I'm here to tell you that I was once in your shoes and if I can do it, you can do it too!

Acknowledgements

I would like to acknowledge my parents, Cynthia and Barry Bartlett who have believed in me and supported me through the good times and the bad.

To my brother Darryl Bartlett who also supported me and played a part in helping me get to where I am today.

To my grandparents Pearl and Harold McGowan and Thomas and Ann Johnson who have been role models that gave me the guts to go for what I want and believe in myself.

To my partners in crime, Amanda McTurk and Donovan Robinson, you two know how much what you have done for me, means to me.

To Dina Vieira whose creativity always amazes me.

To Kathleen Warren who is my number one supporter and cheerleader.

To everyone else who gave me encouragement and support to reach for the stars, I appreciate you!

Foreword

Monique Bartlett is a hard working, dedicated and high performing individual. She spends countless hours working on self-improvement and honing her skills in order to go to the next level.

Kick Start For Weight Loss: 3 Massive Mistakes Professional Women Make That Keep Them Overweight, Exhausted and Stuck On The Diet Treadmill is the result of years of both personal and professional experience. Monique has experienced being overweight and has also helped countless other women reach their ideal weight.

In today's society we tend to be too busy to take responsibility for our own well being. Monique can take you on a journey of your own self development. However, you must be willing to do the work. Treat this book as a workbook, a reference book and pass it on to friends and family. Or better yet, buy them their own copy.

Follow the guidelines in this book and you will reap the rewards of greater happiness, health and confidence.

Gerry Robert
Best Selling Author
The Millionaire Mindset

Table Of Contents

"Take the first step in faith. You don't have to see the whole staircase, just take the first step."

~**Martin Luther King Jr.**

FREE DOWNLOADS

Visit **www.kickstartforweightloss.com/free-tools** for your copy of the forms and worksheets referenced in this book. Please feel free to print copies for your use or to share with your friends, family or colleagues.

My Before and After

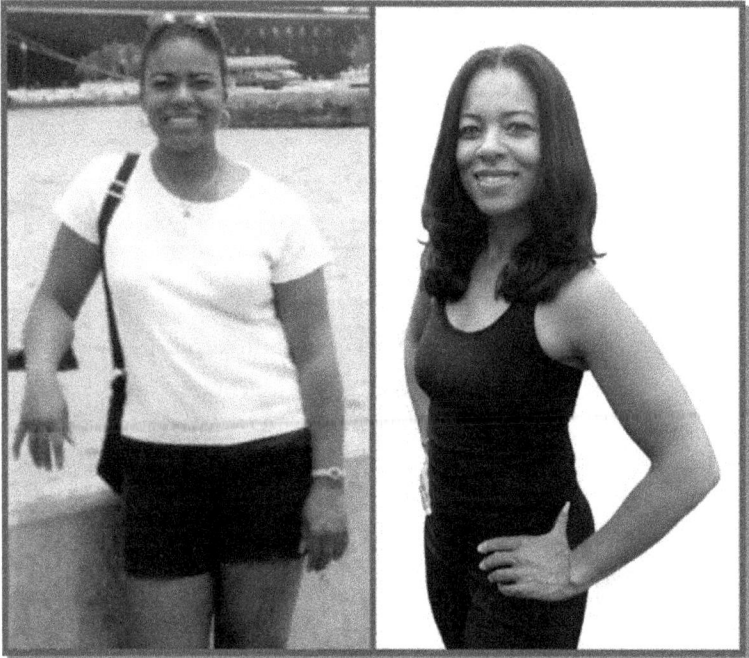

Introduction

Did you know that when women lose weight as part of a group they drop more weight than losing weight alone? The aversion to losing weight while competing with other members of a group can be a good motivator. (Reuters Health)

My name is Monique Bartlett. Welcome to *Kick Start For Weight Loss: 3 Massive Mistakes Professional Women Make That Keep Them Overweight, Exhausted and Stuck On The Diet Treadmill.*

I am an Author, Speaker, Coach and Trainer. I am a former personal trainer who worked at the big gyms and then started my in home personal training business for professional women. I also taught boot camps at several different condos in the Toronto, Ontario area.

You must be thinking, that's great but how did that get you here and what does that mean for me?

Well, when I was a little girl I was very petite. I have pictures of when I was 4 or 5 and to be honest I don't even remember being that tiny. Once puberty hit however, that was all over. By the time I was 13, I was actually the largest of all my friends.

My parents are Jamaican so that means you get served large portions of food and you're expected to eat everything that's put on your plate. The women in my family were overweight but they seemed to be comfortable with the sizes they were. Yet, I felt uncomfortable in my own skin and didn't like what I was seeing in the mirror.

Don't get me wrong, I was actually very active. I played competitive soccer, figure skated and was on the track and volleyball teams in high school, but the problem was I loved to eat. My main problem was my sweet tooth. If it had sugar in it, I wanted to eat it....cookies, cakes, donuts, chocolate bars, candies and the list goes on.

I never really tried to lose weight in high school and then I went away to university and gained the freshman fifteen. You know what I mean, those fifteen pounds that you gain from eating junk food or food from a box or a can because it was inexpensive to buy. With all of the studying and the exams, it was really difficult to eat properly.

This still wasn't enough for me to do anything about losing weight. When I came home from university I moved to Toronto and I was living in a condo that had a gym where they conducted group exercise classes. There was a Pilates class that I wanted to join as I had never done it before but heard that it was great for strengthening without lifting weights. This was perfect for me as I was afraid that lifting weights would make me bulky. I decided to go to the Pilates class and at the first class the instructor asked me if I was pregnant, but I wasn't! That was my a-ha moment.

Through trial and error I wound up losing 30 pounds and was the healthiest and smallest I had ever been in my life. It was a tough road but I did it. It took me about 8 months to lose those 30 pounds but I wasn't in a rush. I went from a size 14 to a size 4. I wanted the weight to come off and stay off and I knew if I followed some drastic diet, that wouldn't happen.

The beauty of it was that people who hadn't seen me for a while didn't recognize me. Half way through my weight loss journey I joined a gym and women would come up to me asking me how I got such defined arms and a toned back. It was at that point that I realized that there were a lot of women struggling with their weight who didn't have the tools they needed to become successful. So I decide to become a personal trainer so that I could give back and help others feel as great as I was feeling.

I worked part time in a few large gyms but then I decided to start my own business doing in home personal training for women. I got a lot of enjoyment helping other women transform themselves and get the results they wanted.

Then it all ended. I was rear ended in a car accident and I couldn't exercise for eight months. I was depressed, had no energy, was in pain, lost all motivation and gained fifteen pounds. I knew I still wanted to help women with their weight loss but I knew that I had to do something else besides personal training.

I was stuck with what I could do to help women get back into shape. I realized that being a personal trainer was great except, that if I couldn't train, I didn't make any money and I could really only help a few women at a time. I had a conversation with a friend of mine and realized that I wanted to write a book. I'd never written anything more than an essay at university so I wasn't sure how I was going to write a book.

I happened to attend a community event and by chance met the publisher of the Toronto Caribbean newspaper. She was looking for a contributor for their fitness section. I wasn't sure why at the time, but I agreed to do a bi-weekly article for the newspaper. That is where the real turn in my life came. I don't usually read my articles once they are published but for some reason I went to the store one day to pick one up and saw an advertisement for the Publish A Book and Grow Rich seminar. I attended that seminar and got amazing ideas for my book.

At that same seminar I also learned about NLP and had found my calling. NLP or Neuro Linguistic Programming is all about how the mind helps create language to change neurology in the brain in order to produce different behavioural results. I realized that these tools could really help me to help others achieve their weight loss goals.

I became an NLP Coach and Hypnosis Trainer and decided to use my coaching and hypnosis skills as the vehicle to make change for professional women who feel stuck, exhausted and are overweight because they put their careers and family first.

NLP helped me realize that it's not just what happens on the outside, it's also about what, negative emotions or limiting decisions we have on the inside. These can cause us to self sabotage ourselves and cause us to fail over and over again. The amount of personal change I have witnessed is unbelievable, not only for myself but for those that I have also been able to help.

The point I'm trying to make is that I know what it's like to be overweight, but I also know what it's like to be healthy. If I can do it, you can too and hopefully this book will help you to reach your a-ha moment. Let me be your tour guide and help you through this journey so you can be, do and have everything you want. It's time for you to maximize your potential and create the results that you desire.

The biggest obstacle you have to overcome in reaching your goals is determining your why. What will motivate you and push you to achieve what you set out to do?

With weight loss it can be any number of things. I know countless amounts of women who say they can't lose weight. They have tried everything already and nothing has worked. They believe that they are just naturally big boned or they say that they're happy with their current weight, even though in reality they're not. The excuses go on and on. So maybe they have tried everything. Maybe they are big boned and maybe they do believe they are happy with how they are currently, however in this day and age more and more people are becoming overweight and obese and putting a strain on the healthcare system.

Do you realize that the current generation is the first generation where many parents are expected to outlive their children because the rate of obesity has grown exponentially?

So if you don't want to lose weight for yourself, you should consider losing weight so you can be around to spend more time with your friends and family. Obesity causes so many diseases that can be prevented, such as heart attacks, strokes, diabetes, high blood pressure, high cholesterol and the list goes on.

To make things a little clearer let me use this analogy. You're afraid of water and someone offers you $25,000 to go into the ocean. For some people $25,000 may be a lot of money but to others it may not be that much. If it's not a lot of money for you, you probably wouldn't even consider it. If it was a lot of money for you, you may actually consider it but your fear would probably take priority and you still wouldn't do it. However imagine you're on a boat and your only child fell in the water and is drowning. You don't know how to swim but you are the only person nearby who can save your precious child's life. I'm pretty sure you would put your child first and jump in the water without even a thought about your own personal safety or your fear.

That's what I mean by a compelling why. So what is your compelling why? Once you figure that out, you'll be able to accomplish anything you set your mind to. Don't get me wrong, there will be hurdles and obstacles along the way. It may take you longer than you thought or you may not lose as much weight as you would like but be proud that you took action and be proud of your accomplishments.

So let's talk about why you bought this book. By the time you reach the end of this book you will learn the answers to the 3 Massive Mistakes   Professional Women Make That Keep Them Overweight, Exhausted and Stuck On The Diet Treadmill:

- ❖ *Why Portion Size Does Matter*
- ❖ *How to Lose Stubborn Belly Fat*
- ❖ *The Solution to Reach Your Ideal Weight*

Chapter One
MASSIVE MISTAKE #3:

Portion Size

Let me ask a question. Do you pay attention to your portion sizes? Well if you don't, let me tell you that your serving size is in direct proportion to your waist line. Even eating too much of healthy foods can lead to weight gain. The problem is that most people perceive portion sizes to be significantly larger than what they are actually meant to be.

It's not only just the portion size, but it's also due to a high amount of calories and low amount of nutrition. People are being overfed but are essentially starving to death. This is because the typical diet is low in fruits, vegetables and whole grains and high in saturated fats, salt and sugar.

Most people also think they take in fewer calories than they actually do. A really great tool to help you keep track of the amount of food you eat is to keep a food journal noting what you eat, when you eat, how much you eat and how you feel when you eat. Are you eating too late? Are you controlling your portion sizes?

It's also important to note how much water you're drinking and if you are eating consistently throughout the day. It can keep you on track by making you aware of what you actually put in your mouth and help you make better choices.

Small changes can result in a big difference in weight loss. See an example of a food journal on the next page.

FOOD JOURNAL				
Food/ Drink	**Description**	**Location**	**Feelings**	**Time**
e.g. type, amount	e.g. amount, cooking method, brand name	e.g. place, people, alone	e.g. hunger, anger, joy	

For a FREE download of the Food Journal go to:
www.kickstartforweightloss.com/free-tools

A great additional tool to use is www.myfitnesspal.com. You can use it online or as an app on your Smartphone. It asks you initial questions to determine your estimated calorie allowance per day. You enter what type of food you eat, how much of it you eat and how much exercise you do in a day. It will subtract the exercise calories from your food calories. It will also show you if you're eating too many carbs, too much sugar or too much salt etc.

It's a really great tool and as long as you're honest with what you write down you will really get to see your eating patterns. You will be amazed to see how much you actually do eat once you write it down. When I first started using it, I couldn't believe how many calories I was consuming during the day. It's just a visual reminder and it actually makes recording what you eat fun.

Portion control is vital to weight management. Limiting portion size reduces calories. The Nutrition Facts panel on a food label is a powerful portion control tool.

Always check the calories and servings per package. You may think a bottle of juice is one serving but when you read the label it's actually two servings. The Nutrition Facts Panel will show the amount of Calories, Fat, Cholesterol, Sodium, Carbohydrates, Sugar etc, for the serving size represented on the label. It is not for the entire box or can unless specified on the package. When the serving size goes up so do the calories, fat, sugar and salt.

If you're not familiar with portion sizes you can use your hand as a guide. Your thumb is equivalent 2 tablespoons, 1 ounce or 30ml. The palm of your hand is equivalent to 3 ounces of meat, fish or poultry or 3 tablespoons of nuts. The size of your fist is equivalent to 1 cup or 2 servings of cooked vegetables and pasta.

Below is an example of a Nutrition Facts Panel.

Nutrition Facts are based on a specific amount of food.

Compare this to the amount you eat.

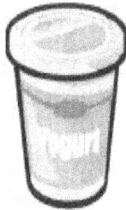

Nutrition Facts	
Per 3/4 cup (175 g)	
Amount	% Daily Value
Calories 160	
Fat 2.5 g	4 %
Saturated 1.5 g + Trans 0 g	8 %
Cholesterol 10 mg	
Sodium 75 mg	3 %
Carbohydrate 25 g	8 %
Fibre 0 g	0 %
Sugars 24 g	
Protein 8 g	
Vitamin A 2 % Vitamin C 0 %	
Calcium 20 % Iron 0 %	

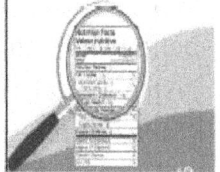

For a FREE download of the Nutrition Facts Panel go to:
www.kickstartforweightloss.com/free-tools

Another really good tip is to measure your bowls and glasses to see how much they actually hold. If you use smaller cups and bowls you'll eat less because your mind thinks you're eating more because the portion sizes look bigger.

When you feel hungry, drink a glass of water first to see if the urge to eat goes away. Thirst is often mistaken for hunger and drinking more water will also help you lose more weight.

The fact of the matter is, the average woman gains about 1 ½ pounds per year during her adult life as her metabolism slows down, muscle loss and bone loss increase, hormones change and stress increases.

It's necessary to eat enough calories to lose weight and not to starve yourself. It's also necessary to get enough sleep to recharge your batteries and get more energy in order to notice your clothes feeling looser.

It's extremely important to eat at regular times. Choose a variety of foods from all food groups, limit sugars and sweets, and reduce the amount of fat you eat. You should include foods high in fibre and protein and limit salt, sugar, alcohol and caffeine.

Eat breakfast daily as breakfast is the most important meal of the day. It keeps your metabolism up and gives you energy to get through the day. Including proteins with your carbs at breakfast will help keep you full and control your appetite throughout the day.

Increase your intake of vegetables and eat protein at every meal. It helps keep you fuller longer and is important for muscle growth and rebuilding muscle, especially when you exercise regularly. Most people want to limit carbs because they feel carbs will make them gain weight. It's actually not the carbs, it's the type of carbs and how much of them you eat. High fibre carbs like brown rice, sweet potatoes or quinoa will help you feel fuller longer so you don't overeat. They're better than the more refined carbs such as white bread, white potatoes and white rice. These carbs get processed in your system and turn into sugar, which is what you don't want.

Eat 5 - 6 times per day. It may sound like a lot but this stabilizes your blood sugar, controls your appetite, increases your metabolism and keeps your energy up. Eat every 3 - 4 hours with 3 average size meals and 2 smaller meals. When you eat too little your body thinks you're starving which causes it to store fat and decrease your metabolism. So when you eat, keep portion sizes in mind and find healthy ways to eat the food you love.

If you're watching what you eat don't think of it as a diet, as a diet sets you up for failure. Eat foods that you enjoy and in moderation as portion size is the key. You don't need to fill your entire plate. Look at it this way, babies only eat until they are satisfied. When they are full they let you know. Only when we get older are we conditioned to finish everything that's put on our plate.

One of the biggest offenders to portion size is eating out. Eating out will cause you to eat more calories as you can't control what ingredients go into or on your food. Not only that, the average portion size in a restaurant is more than double the suggested portion size.

When you eat out with your friends you're also more likely to eat what they're eating and consume extra calories with alcohol. These additional calories add up and slow down your weight loss. When you drink pop, juice, sugary teas and coffees you will consume extra calories which add up to extra pounds. This will occur while you're still watching your food portions and working out regularly. Just because your friend is able to eat additional calories, doesn't mean you can.

Hormones

Before I go any further, it is necessary to make reference to hormones and their effect on weight loss. I will briefly touch upon insulin, leptin, ghrelin, cortisol, estrogen and testosterone.

Insulin is a hormone secreted by the pancreas in response to ingested carbohydrates. Insulin also tells the brain whether or not you should eat and informs the brain about the energy status of your body. When you eat your blood sugar level rises. Your pancreas then releases insulin which in turn tells your brain that you have eaten and to shut off hunger.

The more body fat you have, the more insulin is secreted in response to eating. Insulin resistance can occur if the body doesn't produce enough insulin to maintain a normal blood glucose level causing Type 2 Diabetes. It is possible to regulate your blood sugar levels with food but it is also important to exercise as well.

Leptin is a protein made and released by fat cells. It signals to the body that you have enough energy stored in your fat, so that you should stop eating. It indirectly controls the rate of fat loss as well as both feelings of hunger and satiety. If there is a breakdown in leptin and it doesn't work as it should, it can cause an uncontrollable appetite. One thing you can do is eat a high protein breakfast within 30 minutes of waking in order to regulate your leptin levels.

Ghrelin is a hormone produced in the stomach and pancreas that stimulates hunger. Ghrelin can increase visceral fat especially in the abdominal region and increases the risk of becoming resistant to insulin. High levels of ghrelin stimulate cravings for high calorie foods. One thing you can do to regulate ghrelin is have a high fibre diet.

Cortisol helps regulate blood pressure as well as the body's use of carbohydrates, fats and proteins. Cortisol in itself isn't harmful yet it is increased during times of the flight or fight response and is thus considered to be the stress hormone. Elevated cortisol levels can lower immune function and increase weight gain amongst other things. Cortisol imbalance increases our desire to have carbs and increases abdominal fat. To regulate cortisol you can start by removing stimulating food and drinks such as alcohol and caffeine. You should also get to bed before 11pm.

Estrogen is a steroid hormone that is produced in the ovaries, fat cells and adrenal glands. Estrogen dominance can occur in women for 10 to 15 years starting as early as age 35. Estrogen dominance has been linked to cancer, infertility, ovarian cysts and acceleration of aging. A high fibre diet and increasing cruciferous vegetables such as broccoli as well as omega 3 fatty acids, can help to balance estrogen.

Testosterone is a steroid hormone that is produced in the testes in men and in the cells of the ovaries and adrenal glands in women. It is responsible for energy balance, increasing muscle mass and bone mass. It also impacts glucose, insulin and fat metabolism. Testosterone can be regulated by removing sugar and processed foods and increasing resistance training. It is also important to reduce stress and improve your sleeping habits.

I have only briefly touched on hormones but there is so much more to them. If you find that you are having difficulty losing weight especially around the mid section and are tired and seem to be constantly hungry, then perhaps you may have a hormone imbalance and should consider making hormonal balance a priority.

Chapter Two
MASSIVE MISTAKE #2:

Spot Training to Lose Stubborn Belly Fat

Have you ever tried to spot train and didn't get great results?

In researching this book I interviewed professional women and asked them which one body part they would most like to lose weight from if they had the choice. The overwhelming answer was the belly/stomach/love handles. They want to look great in a bathing suit and use a flat stomach as their benchmark.

Even though most women would like to lose their belly for cosmetic reasons, it's really important to lose belly fat to help reduce the risk of disease. Diseases such as type 2 diabetes, sleep apnea, heart disease, high blood pressure and some research has also shown even certain cancers.

So, how do you lose stubborn belly fat? The answer is by increasing your metabolism and burning fat. Ultimately you need to strength train and increase your cardio for your entire body. When most women think about strength training, they imagine that it will cause big and bulky muscles. This idea could not be further from the truth.

Male testosterone which is the primary cause of muscle development is 10 - 30 times higher than females. On average, women carry about double the amount of fat as men. This is due to the effects of estrogen which is involved in the storage of body fat, causing women to have a tougher time losing belly fat.

A woman's premenstrual cycle usually comes with fluid retention and cravings for sweets which can also cause temporary weight gain. Also, when a woman goes through pregnancy there are a lot of biological changes that take place. There is an increase in body fat levels as it is necessary for fetal development. This causes appetite and food cravings to increase and metabolism to slow down.

To maximize fat loss, the focus should always be exercise that increases lean muscle mass and burns calories. Strength training helps promote fat loss and is important in long term weight management. Strength training can sculpt the body in many ways. You can add muscle mass, increase strength and improve muscle tone. Your main goal should be to tone and shape your muscles. At some point you may find that you've developed a little more muscle than you like. Just simply take some time off training or reduce your workout intensity.

Strength training increases your metabolism, burns extra calories, and once you build up muscle it also burns more calories at rest. That being said, spot reducing is not effective in reducing fat in any one particular body area. You can do all of the crunches you like but the truth is that you can't spot train by doing abdominal exercises in order to lose the belly fat.

The best option is to exercise your larger muscle groups so that you burn more calories over all. Once you start to reduce the fat, you can target the abs and help tone the muscles to get a tighter stomach.

Increasing your muscle mass will not necessarily cause the scale to move immediately but it will decrease your inches. 5 pounds of muscle and 5 pounds of fat weigh the same; however lean muscle mass takes up less space.

Dr. Natasha Turner ND, Founder of Clear Medicine Wellness Boutique says, *"This is my formula for weight loss – hormonal balance plus the difference in calories (calories in through diet – and out through exercise) equals lasting weight loss and the ability to lose weight. So many of us believe we can get healthy by losing weight. However, the truth is we must be healthy in order to lose weight. Since hormones are the key to controlling our appetite and stimulating our metabolism, then achieving and maintaining hormonal balance plays an essential role in lasting fat loss. Yes, diet and exercise are important, but so are sleeping well, reducing toxin exposure, maintaining healthy liver function, optimizing digestion, limiting stress, having the right mindset and conquering inflammation. All of these factors can influence our hormonal activity – and weight loss success – in truly dramatic ways."*

Expect to see results every 3 - 4 weeks. It only takes your body about 4 weeks to get used to a workout routine and once that happens you're bound to hit a plateau. You will need to change up your workout routine so your body will begin to keep dropping fat and lose weight.

That's why it's important to strength train as strength training can break through a plateau faster than any other method. If you're not sure that strength training is right for you, begin with simple body weight exercises such as push ups, sit ups, burpees or planks. Once you feel you are ready for something more then you can begin a more intense strength training routine.

If you're really unsure where to start, find a coach or a trainer who can help get you started. If you aren't looking for a long term commitment I would suggest a minimum of 3 sessions. This will give you enough information and an initial boost of confidence to get you started on the right track. If you can afford it though, it would be a good idea to get a coach at least twice a week for the first 90 days. This will help you form good habits and you will get better and faster results.

Louyse Vigneault who is a Fitness Instructor says, *"Nutrition is the main part of health but you need a mixture of cardio, weights and flexibility so you can build muscle and burn calories at rest."*

Be realistic in what you can and cannot do on your way to weight loss success. Don't commit to working out 5 days a week if you know you can only do 3. Even though 3 workouts are more than you did before, you will feel as if you failed if you do not complete the 5 workouts you committed to completing.

Your time is valuable and you want to make the most of it. Work, family and social commitments can compete for your time and energy leaving you with very little time and energy to eat right and exercise. However, an exercise program can provide you with more energy, confidence, stamina, self esteem and greater productivity.

Many women have tried and failed at exercise programs in the past. Whatever forced you off track last time will more than likely cause you to get off track again. I believe it was Albert Einstein who said *"The definition of insanity is doing the same thing over and over again expecting different results."*

In order to get a different result it is important to establish and set boundaries. Change up meals, schedule workouts like you would a doctor or dentist appointment and make losing weight a priority.

Life eventually starts to take over and it is almost inevitable that you will lose your motivation as other things start to become more important. At this point it's time for you to take a step back and remember why you initially began this journey. What was your goal? What was your pain? You need to remember why you started and keep the end in sight.

Get your head back in the game. Are you hanging around with like-minded people? Do you have a workout buddy to keep you accountable? Remember to keep it fun and eat foods that you like but everything in moderation. Pick activities that you enjoy doing even if it's just taking your dog out for a walk or going swimming. Every little bit helps. Don't deprive yourself from what you enjoy but give yourself intermittent rewards.

If you were on track from Monday to Friday go ahead and have that slice of cake you enjoy on Saturday (just don't eat the entire cake!) If there's a particular dress size you're aiming for at the end of your initial 90 days, go ahead and buy yourself a goal outfit and hang it where you will see it every day so it can motivate you. Imagine how good you're going to look in it. Imagine all of the confidence you're going to have wearing it and the compliments you will receive when your friends and family see you in it.

Once you get into the outfit go out for a night on the town. Your compelling why is what will keep pushing you to reach your goal. Only you know if you're sick and tired of being sick and tired. Only you know that it doesn't feel good to be out of breath climbing a set of stairs. Only you know how it feels to give yourself insulin shots every day because you have diabetes related to weight issues. Only you know what type of life your children would have to live and how devastated they would be to have to live their life without you.

Whatever your motivating factor is, remember, it doesn't matter if you have a few bad days or even a few bad weeks. Believe that you can do it and you will become the new and improved you.

Losing weight and getting healthy is no small feat. If it was easy everyone would be able to do it. You have to take responsibility for your actions and be willing to go the extra mile. Ultimately your attitude determines your actions. You've got to focus your attention on the long term goal but it's important to give yourself short term goals as well. If you had to wait until the end of your 90 day goal to really celebrate and reward yourself you would give up in no time.

Starting with smaller more manageable steps will keep you on track and will motivate you to push you through until the end. Get rid of all your excuses and set your priorities. If you have to wake up an hour earlier to fit some exercise into your day do it. If you have to stay up an hour later because you had a crazy day and had to eat a little later than normal do it.

Don't go to bed with a full stomach. Give your food the chance to digest for at least an hour. You'll be able to sleep better and your body won't want to store those extra fat calories.

It's up to you to get the job done. If you have an injury that doesn't mean you stop doing everything, work around it. Find out what works for you. Don't listen to the little voice in your head telling you to give up. If you don't succeed at the first try that just means this particular way doesn't work for you. Figure out what will work for you and start again.

Get a mentor, a coach or trainer. Be accountable not just to yourself but to someone else who wants you to succeed, probably more than you want to see yourself succeed. If you don't have anyone available in your immediate circle go to **www.moniquebartlett.com** and register for a free 30 minute strategy session and let me help you get on track.

You may not think you can do it but you really can. I have walked a similar path and it wasn't easy for me, yet I had the passion and desire because I knew I needed to make a change. I had my good days and bad days. It's not how long it takes you to reach your goal, it's the plan you choose to get you to it.

See your family physician before beginning any exercise program and be prepared for aches, pains and stiffness in your first few weeks. Regularly take your measurements and monitor improvements with duration and reps in your exercise program.

Take before and after pictures so you can monitor your progress and really see the changes that are happening with your body. You will be surprised at how quickly changes can happen that you don't notice initially. You will also notice that you will have an increase in energy and endurance. You will feel so much better about yourself and like what you see in the mirror.

Use the chart on the following page as a guide. Track your measurements and physical strength. For each of the exercises in the physical strength column track how many you can do of each exercise in 2 minutes.

Client Name_____

Date_____

Measured Results	Starting Results	After 4 Weeks	Change	Ultimate Goal	
Weight					
Body Fat Percentage					
Height					
Circumference Measurements					
Left Arm					
Right Arm					
Chest					
Waist					
Hips					
Upper Left Thigh					
Upper Right Thigh					
Left Calf					
Right Calf					
Front & Back Picture					
Physical Strength					
Push Ups					
Sit Ups					
Jumping Jacks					

For a FREE download of the Measurement Tracking Guide
go to:
www.kickstartforweightloss.com/free-tools

Chapter Three
MASSIVE MISTAKE #1:

Relying Only On Diet and Exercise

Do you feel as if you are constantly trying to lose weight but the results never seem to be permanent?

The reason for this is that food doesn't cause you to be overweight, your thoughts do. Being overweight is actually not the problem; it's the solution to family abuse, stress, a dead end job, trauma, bad relationships, sadness, dehydration and sleep deprivation.

Your body protects you with fat. That's why you need to create a mind/body connection. What is a mind/body connection? It's being able to train your mind to get you out of old patterns of behaviour that aren't serving you, so you can set new ones.

It probably took you a lifetime to accumulate all of your fattening habits. Your routine is producing the results you get. Treating the symptoms will never change anything, as you will always fall back into your past behaviours. You have to get to the root of the problem.

Dr. Justine Blainey, a Chiropractor who owns the Justine Blainey Wellness Centre, took a complaint to the Human Rights Commission so that girls could play hockey with boys and won. Dr. Blainey says, *"In order to lose weight you not only need to find the root of the problem but look to the nervous system. Your health is your responsibility. Taking care of your health is not selfish. The decisions we make today affect our families. If you need someone to keep you on track hire a coach because we tend to start and then we quit."*

You think with your conscious mind but your actions are controlled by your unconscious mind. What is your conscious mind? Your conscious mind is your thinking mind. It chooses your thoughts and accepts and rejects ideas. It is the part of your mind that you hear talking in your head all the time.

The unconscious mind controls your actions and the body. It has no ability to reject and controls feelings and emotions. It is what you use in your daily acts. You no longer have to think about it, you can do it in your sleep. Your beliefs are stored in your unconscious mind. It doesn't know the difference between what's real and imagined.

There are specific thoughts and feelings in your unconscious mind that have an impact on your eating patterns. Being overweight is a symptom of these thoughts and feelings. The second you tell your mind you're on a diet you go into a paradigm of "I can't." Instead, say that you can, but you choose not to.

You need to eliminate the following words from your vocabulary: if, doubt, don't, I don't think, I don't have time, maybe, I'm afraid of, I don't believe, but.

Answer the following questions:

1. What's going on in your mind right now? What are you saying to yourself about your weight?

   _____
   _____
   _____
   _____

2. What's the message in your head? Do you have positive or negative thoughts?

   _____
   _____
   _____
   _____

3. What's your intention for food? Is it for nourishment or to ease emotional issues?

_____

_____

_____

_____

4. What's missing in your life right now? How can you fill the void without using food?

_____

_____

_____

_____

5. What are your eating triggers? Are they boredom, stress, anger, sadness, fear, hurt, guilt, shame, depression?

_____

_____

_____

_____

6. What are the benefits of eating vs. not eating? What secondary gain do you get from eating? Are you punishing yourself or someone else?

_____

_____

_____

_____

Logic tells you that you need to lose weight. You want to feel better, look better, have more confidence, more energy and more self control.

The reality is that it's not just what you're eating; it's what's eating you. Change your focus from a diet, to why your body wants to be fat. You know you shouldn't eat what you're eating, but you do it anyway.

Lori Kennedy who is a Board Certified Practical Holistic Nutritionist and owner of WOW Weight Loss says, *"You can lose weight but that doesn't mean that you're healthy. Learn how to manage life such as daily challenges with food, emotions and understand their triggers. You get to make the choice. Learn to implement life changing habits. Ask yourself how open you are to make changes. Build from your comfort level. Do one thing at a time."*

Move towards the good things and away from the bad things. What are your current thoughts about your body and your weight? Do you wonder how you will reach your goal? The unconscious mind solves the puzzle. Change your mindset and change your life.

In order to change your habits you need to understand the 4 Stages of Learning which are on the following page.

4 Stages of Learning

❖ Unconscious Incompetence – you don't know that you don't know how to do something. This is the stage of ignorance before your learning begins.
❖ Conscious Incompetence – you know that you don't know how to do it. This is where your learning begins and you will make some mistakes.
❖ Conscious Competence – you know that you can do it. You are still learning and are a bit uncomfortable and self conscious because you have to think about what to do next.
❖ Unconscious Competence – you know it and it becomes a natural part of you. You only have to think about it when something alerts you to it.

Now that you know the 4 Stages of Learning, you should also know that the mind has between 60,000 - 90,000 thoughts per day. 96% of those thoughts are repeated every day.

You've got to start paying attention to the thoughts in your mind **right now**. If it's good or bad, you need to decide how to react to the message. You need to install new beliefs in order to stop self sabotage. On the next page you will learn 5 signs of self sabotaging behaviour.

5 Signs of Self-Sabotaging Behaviour

- ❖ Focusing on what is not working or not right.
- ❖ Being stuck in fear.
- ❖ Feeling as if you have no value.
- ❖ Comparing yourself to others.
- ❖ Feeling as if you have no purpose.

Start stating positive new conscious thoughts and your mind will begin to start processing that information and store them as new beliefs. Get the new information you need, not what you already know. Lifestyle change can be overwhelming for everyone. You just need to be ready to commit to change.

Successful people make quick decisions so just decide and start to take action. Start today; there's no time better than the present. Learning a new strategy to get you from a negative emotion to a positive emotion will benefit your success. In order to do this you need to get your mindset right. In order to create a positive mindset, you need to understand the 3 requisites for change which you will learn on the following page.

3 Requisites for Change

❖ Clean up your past patterns such as negative emotions and limiting decisions.
❖ Focus on what you want.
❖ Dedicate your resources of time, money and energy towards what you want and **TAKE ACTION!**

In order to get you where you need to be, you need to know where you have come from. There are currently negative and positive beliefs that are creating both physical and emotional changes in your behaviour. These beliefs create the programs that run in your mind. These programs are usually formed somewhere between the ages of 0 - 5 years old, which run unconsciously in the background of your mind.

At this point we are programmed to think like the people we are surrounded by. These habits are the ideas that have been programmed into the unconscious mind over and over again. These programs can create self sabotaging behaviours and can cause you to feel bad about how you look in the mirror or cause you to use food as an emotional crutch amongst many other things. These beliefs and habits determine whether you are on the side of cause or effect; which you will learn on the following page.

Cause & Effect

❖ You need to train your mind and decide whether you are living on the cause or effect side of the equation.

❖ If you're on the side of cause, you are in control. You influence and take responsibility for everything that happens in your life.

❖ If you're on the side of effect, you live your life based on excuses of why you can't affect or control what you say or do.

❖ Stop arguing for your limitations.

❖ Develop new skills in order to create change.

❖ Something will always test you, how bad do you want success?

❖ Decide it's possible.

You have great intentions and enthusiasm when you begin to lose weight, but within a short time you lose interest due to frustration, personal issues, discomfort and other factors.

You need to get rid of your limiting beliefs. Get rid of any competing thoughts, feelings, beliefs or behaviours that are not supporting you. Imagine the life you will be enjoying in your new future. What are you doing? Who are you with? How do you feel? What is your current mindset?

Thinking about weight loss goals you didn't accomplish in your past does not help your present or your future. I once heard Oprah Winfrey say this quote and it really struck a chord with me, *"Forgiveness is giving up the hope that the past could've been any different."* You can't keep dwelling on why you haven't accomplished your goal. It only holds space in your mind. What are you most afraid of that is getting in the way? You need to act as if you have already lost the weight you wanted to lose, even if your weight is currently not where you want to be.

Visualize the body you want to have. See, feel, imagine yourself being in the body you want when your mind is calm, powerful and relaxed. Visualize the fitness level you want for yourself. See yourself accomplishing the fitness goals you'd like to achieve. Get a real sense of what it will be like to achieve your goal. Compare where you are right now and why you want the change.

You're now at the point where your clothes don't fit, you don't have the energy to do what you want to do, your back is aching, your blood pressure is skyrocketing, your cholesterol is high or your doctor told you need to start exercising.

Realize that you can't attract your perfect weight if you feel bad about your body now. If you can't imagine what you want, how will you get there? Your brain can't distinguish reality from imagination. Get a picture of what you want to look like. Cut a picture out of a magazine or use a picture of you when you were happier with your weight.

Just make sure your weight loss goal is realistic and achievable. If your goal is not attainable and not realistic it will not motivate you. It's realistic to expect to lose 6 - 8 pounds a month. It's not realistic to expect to lose 20 pounds or more a month.

Do you have limiting beliefs about what your body can look like? Buy a dress in the size you want to be in and hang it in a prominent spot where it will motivate you and be a powerful incentive. High level Olympic athletes use visualization to help them achieve top performances. Why can't you? What pain are you forced to endure if you stay at your current weight right now?

It's time to start setting boundaries that align with your values and beliefs, in order for you to start on your journey to reach your ideal weight.

Boundary Settings

If you do not set boundaries you will get off track very easily. Set a course for growth and align your resources. You need to set boundaries and know your current values and beliefs in order to reach your goal. Without setting your boundaries others will take advantage and force you off track in order to get what they want.

- ❖ You will receive an external request for time, money or energy.
- ❖ Ask yourself these three questions:
- ❖ Do I have it?
- ❖ Am I willing to give it?
- ❖ Under what conditions?
- ❖ Negotiate your terms and set consequences if you do not stay within the realm of your boundaries.

Values

Values are the things a person considers most important.

❖ These are things such as career, family, relationships, personal growth, health and fitness, spirituality and more.

❖ Even if you don't realize it, your values drive your actions. They run all of your beliefs and your beliefs run all of your behaviours.

❖ Your values also drive your goals. Without knowing our values it's difficult to reach your goals.

❖ The way you use your time and money shows what you value.

You realize that you should exercise more and eat better in order to lose weight. However, there is obviously a gap between knowing and doing; otherwise there wouldn't be so many women who are overweight.

The issue seems to be with the motivation or the method that you take when initiating weight loss. You're not happy with your present level of fitness and the way your body looks but you're not willing to make the necessary changes. Change is difficult, but you need to set up the proper framework for success.

A certain level of planning is needed before you begin a weight loss program. You wouldn't take a trip without figuring out where you're going first or putting the address in your GPS, so why would you want to lose weight without planning for it first? Commit to overcoming your fear of failure and force yourself to take some risks.

Losing weight can be a challenge on a good day. You may be constantly exhausted, unhappy, unmotivated and feel unattractive. You may feel as if your clothes are a little too tight and you have a little bit of extra fat around your waist. When you're stressed, depressed or have back or joint pain, it's even more difficult.

Even losing just 10% of your body weight can make a huge difference to your overall health. It can lower your blood pressure, lower your cholesterol and even prevent heart disease. Not losing weight can cause you to feel uncomfortable in your own skin, cause depression or even cause stress in your personal and professional life.

The real key to weight loss is to begin with a clean slate to get you to your goal. You need to learn new strategies and get new tools in order to lose weight.

You need to think of food as a means to satisfy hunger and not as a means to relieve stress or avoid negative emotions. The problem is that when you're busy you don't address your emotional eating. You may tend to use food as a crutch. You may use food to mask pain, hurt, anger, depression, punishment, guilt, anxiety, escape and fear. You may also skip meals or be a poor eater.

You may unconsciously eat at your desk, in your car or watching TV. You may not drink enough water and dehydration makes you hungry. You may use food as a reward system. You may not address your stress and stress is the number one cause of emotional eating. You may do too much and don't know how to ask for help or say no.

You may keep hearing your parents tell you to eat everything on your plate. You may be overweight, stressed out and unhappy. You may have tried to lose weight before but were unsuccessful, so you figure why bother? You may be afraid that you will keep failing in your weight loss journey and lose confidence in yourself.

You need to figure out what problems you are facing that are keeping you overweight. You need to make the decision and be committed to seeing it through. Getting rid of negative thoughts and taking positive action for 90 days will create a new habit and will create a new behaviour for life.

Answer the following questions:

1. What is important to you about losing weight?
   _____
   _____
   _____
   _____

2. What does your ideal body look like?
   _____
   _____
   _____
   _____

3. What are you willing to do to get it?
   _____
   _____
   _____
   _____

4. What do you see/hear/feel when you imagine being at your ideal weight?
   _____
   _____
   _____
   _____

Create your vision for what you want. Build your vision into your unconscious to change your outside world. Focus on what you want. Are you moving closer to or farther away from it?

Have short term and long term goals. Pick a date by which you want to achieve them and write them down. Look at them every day. The unconscious mind will tell the conscious mind the right thing to do. Focus on what you need to do to hit each goal.

1. What do you need to change in your life in order to reach your ideal weight right now?

   _____

   _____

   _____

   _____

2. What do you need more of: time, money or energy?

   _____

   _____

   _____

   _____

3. What can you measure on a weekly basis to make sure you're on track? Inches, pounds?

   _____

   _____

   _____

   _____

4. What will keep you focused on reaching your ideal weight?

_____

_____

_____

_____

5. How do you feel about yourself right now? How would you like to feel about yourself in the future?

_____

_____

_____

_____

6. How do your clothes fit? Are they too tight, a little snug?

_____

_____

_____

_____

7. How long have you had your goal and done nothing about it?

_____

_____

_____

_____

8. What is stopping you from **being** what you want, **doing** what you want and **having** what you want right now?

_____

_____

_____

_____

9. Are you willing to take a risk to get from where you are right now to where you want to be?

_____

_____

_____

_____

Focus on losing body fat or inches rather than weight loss. Focus on positive changes in daily eating and new exercise habits. If your goal doesn't scare you and excite you at the same time, your goal isn't big enough.

The first thing you need to do is define your who, what, where, when and why.

1. What are you going to do to reach your goal?

_____

_____

_____

_____

2. What date are you going to do it by?

_____

_____

_____

_____

3. Why do you want reach your ideal weight?

_____

_____

_____

_____

4. Who will support you and help you reach your goal?

_____

_____

_____

_____

5. Where will you do it in order to maximize your results?

_____

_____

_____

_____

SMART Goals

The most important element is your why. Without this, the rest doesn't matter. If your why isn't compelling enough you will never achieve your goal. Your why will help you get from where you are now, to actually achieving your dream. Your why will make your goal so compelling that you can only achieve it.

In order to get a compelling why, start with a SMART Goal. **A SMART Goal is Specific, Measurable, Achievable, Realistic and Timed**. It will align your habits with your goals and give you an action plan. It will allow you to set boundaries and keep you on the right path.

If you want to achieve your goals you are usually physically capable of achieving them. It comes down to how badly you really want them. You need to stick to the program long enough to enjoy the benefits. Most people associate pain with exercise and hate every second of it. Instead, they should consider the pain of imagining their life without it. Associate more pleasure with getting your goals, than the pain of not getting your goals.

Consistency is the key to success and radical changes are not necessary. Small consistent changes can bring out the best, long lasting results. Establish small goals on the way to your large goal. The small steps to success will build confidence and self esteem. This instills belief that you'll make it to your ultimate goal. If you make a healthy lifestyle part of your routine like brushing your teeth or taking a shower, it will become a habit and seeing results will keep you motivated.

Goals reinforce the fact that what you want is real and achievable. Write down the goals you would like to achieve. It's a great way to keep you motivated. Have a deadline that can't be adjusted.

Have a goal of completing an event. For example a walk, run, triathlon, cycling, hiking, etc. Once the event is completed you can't take that away. You can always say that you did it and will have the photos and memories forever. When you're training for a purpose it makes it easier to stick to your program. If an event is not possible consider something like, being able to run on the treadmill for an hour without stopping by a set date.

Use the chart on page 54 to assist you with setting your SMART Goal.

In order to make your goal **Specific**, ask yourself; *"What do I want to do?"* For example, you can make your goal be I want to weigh 130 pounds. It's specific enough yet also simple enough for you to remember. Write your specific goal:

_____

_____

_____

_____

Make your goal **Measurable** by asking yourself: *"How much do I want to lose and how often will I exercise?"* For example, I want to lose 2 inches off my hips, 2 inches off my waist, 5% body fat and 15 pounds overall. I will accomplish this by walking 2 days a week and going to the gym to do strength training 3 days a week. Write your specific goal:

_____

_____

_____

_____

To make your goal **Attainable** ask yourself: *"How will I do it?"* In this case it is important to state your goal as if you have already achieved it. For example, I am excited that I am lifting weights 3 days a week as it makes me feel stronger and healthier. Write your attainable goal:

_____

_____

_____

_____

To make your goal **Realistic** ask yourself: *"Can I do it?"* If you really do not believe you can accomplish it and if it is not in the best interest of you or others who are supporting you during your goal, then do not do it. For example, I will train at the gym 2 days a week on my own for an hour and 1 day a week with my personal trainer. Write your realistic goal:

_____

_____

_____

_____

To make your goal **Timed** ask yourself: *"When will I do it by?"* Make sure your goal is framed in the language of what you want. For example, I am 130 pounds by December 31. Write your timed goal:

_____

_____

_____

_____

An example of a SMART Goal would be:

I am celebrating the fact that it is December 31, 2xxx and I am 130 pounds. I have lost 15 pounds and 5% body fat, now that I have been strength training at the gym 3 days a week on my own and 1 day a week with my personal trainer.

Your SMART Goal needs to be stated positively and towards what you want. You need to make sure that you are doing this because you want to, not because someone else wants it for you.

Write your SMART Goal:

_____
_____
_____
_____
_____
_____
_____
_____

			What do I want to do?
S	Specific		
M	Measureable		How much and how often will I do it?
A	Attainable		How will I do it?
R	Realistic		Can I do it?
T	Timely		When will I do it?

My SMART Goal

Name: _____   Date: _____

For a FREE download of the SMART Goal chart go to:
www.kickstartforweightloss.com/free-tools

Have a support system with positive people who want you to succeed. Let them support you on your good days and not so good days. Make sure they will keep you accountable and help you realize when you reach your goal.

If you don't have all the resources you need to be successful, make sure you find out where you can get them. Know what secondary gain you will be experiencing if you do not reach your goal.

1. What will you lose if you don't reach your goal?

_____

_____

_____

_____

2. What will you gain if you do reach your goal?

_____

_____

_____

_____

Keep your SMART Goal on the mirror in your bathroom so you can see it every day and it will help to keep you motivated. Writing everything down can lead you on your roadmap to success. Write down action steps that are moving you closer to achieving your goals. Let your accountability partner know when you are accomplishing your action steps.

Action Step Guide

Write down 3 action steps weekly that will move you closer to your goal.

Contact your accountability partner weekly when you complete your steps.

Goal	Week 1 - Contacted Partner ☐	Week 2 - Contacted Partner ☐
	1	1
	2	2
	3	3
	Week 3 - Contacted Partner ☐	Week 4 - Contacted Partner ☐
	1	1
	2	2
	3	3
	Week 5 - Contacted Partner ☐	Week 6 - Contacted Partner ☐
	1	1
	2	2
	3	3
	Week 7 - Contacted Partner ☐	Week 8 - Contacted Partner ☐
	1	1
	2	2
	3	3
	Week 9 - Contacted Partner ☐	Week 10 - Contacted Partner ☐
	1	1
	2	2
	3	3
	Week 11 - Contacted Partner ☐	Week 12 - Contacted Partner ☐
	1	1
	2	2
	3	3

For a FREE download of the Action Step Guide go to:
www.kickstartforweightloss.com/free-tools

Chapter 4

Weight Loss and Hypnosis

Did you know that hypnosis is a great tool to use in order to help you in reach your ideal weight? Hypnosis can assist you in changing your beliefs and if you can change your beliefs then you can change your results. It is about consciously deciding to change your thoughts to support the results you want to have in your life. By learning to communicate with your unconscious mind, you can provide the future you want tomorrow.

Hypnosis can be extremely effective if the situation is correct. How you interpret the words and feelings that come to you determines how you feel. If those words and feelings become positive you will receive positive results. Do you have beliefs that are currently holding you back?

Hypnosis allows you to focus on what you want so you can get what you want. The truth is that all hypnosis is self hypnosis. You should not expect to feel hypnotised, it is a normal state of relaxation. Hypnosis will not make you do anything you don't want to do. You only accept suggestions that are given that are consistent with your internal values and beliefs. If you were asked to stand up you would probably do that, but if you were asked to jump off the CN Tower without a parachute, I'm sure you wouldn't do that.

At various times throughout a typical day without even realizing it, we go into a natural state of hypnosis. Day dreaming or forgetting how you got home from work are forms of hypnosis. A hypnotherapist is the guide and you are the tourist searching for that state of mind.

Hypnosis is completely safe and is a heightened state of awareness. You are in complete control at all times. You can come out of the hypnotic state at any time. The hypnotherapist never has control over you. You will remember everything, just as if you were in a normal state of mind.

The hypnotic state gives you 10,000 times more focus. You probably don't realize it but you are already in trance about 85% of your day. Hypnosis is used to help you get what you need. It is best for people who are intelligent, creative and like to be in control, as hypnosis is the ultimate display of control.

The mind creates realistic thoughts and the body responds. It can transfer you from a problem to a solution. It takes 10 times more energy to stay stuck than to transform, so why continue to stay stuck?

You know you need to lose weight, but something is holding you back. The majority of weight issues are due to deep underlying rooted issues that you may not even be aware of. These are things you may not have been able to address at an earlier point in your life or you didn't have the tools to get you to where you needed to be.

By focusing on what you want, you are sending a message to your unconscious mind to find every opportunity to move you towards your goal. If you consistently think of yourself at your ideal weight and keep reinforcing that with your beliefs and behaviours you will make greater advances to reach your ideal weight.

How Effective Is Hypnosis?

Results of Comparative Study
by *American Health Magazine:*

Psychoanalysis:
38% recovery after 600 sessions

Behavior Therapy:
72% recovery after 22 sessions

Hypnotherapy:
93% recovery after 6 sessions

❖ Psychoanalysis or psychiatry – uses dreams or fantasies and interprets the information to create an insight into the resolution of the problem.

❖ Behaviour therapy – uses classical conditioning e.g. Pavlov's theory.

Imagine a slimmer, healthier you that overcomes unhealthy food cravings and minimizes all the bad carbohydrates, sugars, starches, and trans-fats.

A hypnosis weight loss program can help you lose weight. You will be highly focused and more responsive to ideas about behavioral changes, in eating habits. This provides a natural and quick and easy way to reach your ideal weight.

Hypnosis can be used to help you become aware of why you overeat. It's about training your mind to think about food in a different way or you will never be successful reaching your ideal weight.

Hypnosis uses techniques such as visualisation in order to assist you to take control of your eating habits and enjoy the benefits of healthy eating. This often involves uncovering an initial event from early childhood which triggered this behaviour pattern. This empowers you to make long term positive changes to your life without the need for willpower. In hypnosis you will feel relaxed and comfortable although you remain in total control of your actions.

Hypnosis enables immediate change of habits and patterns. It causes a physiological change to occur in the brain, which makes it more receptive to suggestion for positive change. When you know why you are doing something, it makes it easier for you to change it.

With hypnosis, there is no longer a battle between the mind and body. Doing healthy, active things that make reaching your ideal weight pleasurable, and making healthy choices, makes it easier to lose weight rather than feeling deprived or victimized by a strict diet and exercise program.

Kick Start For Weight Loss Bootcamp™

If you're interested in learning more about how hypnosis can help you with your weight loss and find better tools to get you out of your comfort zone, register for my **Kick Start For Weight Loss Bootcamp™.** This 6 month online course is comprised of:

- ❖ 6 Month Online Program
- ❖ Step By Step Personalized Plans
- ❖ How To Read Nutrition Labels
- ❖ How Hormones Affect Weight Loss
- ❖ Learn About Fibre, Carbs And Supplements In Detail
- ❖ How To Grocery Shop And Set Appropriate Goals
- ❖ How To Eat On The Go
- ❖ How Stress And Sleep Affect Weight Loss
- ❖ Interactive Monthly Group Calls
- ❖ Private Facebook Group
- ❖ 1 on 1 Coaching Calls
- ❖ Downloadable Worksheets
- ❖ Ongoing Email Support
- ❖ Go to **www.moniquebartlett.com/workshops** to find out more information.

You will also receive a complimentary 30 minute discovery session which will help you to determine if you're really ready to make this change for yourself right now.

FREE DOWNLOADS

Visit **www.kickstartforweightloss.com/free-tools** for your copy of the forms and worksheets referenced in this book. Please feel free to print copies for your use or to share with your friends, family or colleagues.

Chapter 5

Taking Action

Keep looking for inspiration. Get to the point where regular exercise and better eating habits are a way of life for you. Live a healthier and happier life. There so many more possibilities that have now opened up to you. The trick is to continue on your journey to health and happiness. If you can help at least one person accomplish the same success in their journey as you, then that is an even greater success. I would love to hear your success story.

E-mail me at: **monique@moniquebartlett.com**

Let me know how your journey has been. Send me your before and after photos and you will placed in a draw for a complimentary 60 minute strategy session.

If you're struggling with being able to get to your after picture, consider this the opportunity for you to reach out to me. Remember, I've been there. My goal is to help 1,000,000 professional women who are overweight, exhausted and stuck on the diet treadmill to reach their ideal weight and feel good about themselves again.

It's up to you to make sure that life doesn't get in the way again. Get an accountability partner or ongoing support to make sure your routine doesn't become old and that you don't get stuck back in old bad habits.

Find 3 new ways to improve your current routine or habits; whether that's adding 3 new exercises to your exercise routine for the next 90 days or adding 3 new foods to your menu that you've never tried before. Whatever you choose make sure it's something you can stick to.

Determine what other maintenance needs you have. Is it speaking with your health coach on a regular basis? Is it working out with your trainer 1 or 2 days a week? It can be anything that you know will help keep you on track. Stay focused on your results. Don't sway from all of the gains you have made.

The goal is for you to create freedom, empowerment and self awareness. Remember, you can't solve a problem with the level of thinking that created it. Take a few minutes to answer the questions on the following page.

Self Awareness Questions

1. What is most important to you about your health/weight?

   _____

   _____

   _____

   _____

2. How will you know when you've reached your goal? What is essential for you to see, hear, feel or learn to know that you have achieved your outcome?

   _____

   _____

   _____

   _____

3. What has to happen for you to take action now?

   _____

   _____

   _____

   _____

4. What does an ideal weight mean to you?

   _____

   _____

   _____

   _____

5. What do you like most about your body right now?

    _____

    _____

    _____

    _____

6. What do you like least about your body right now?

    _____

    _____

    _____

    _____

7. What is the biggest challenge you have with reaching your ideal weight?

    _____

    _____

    _____

    _____

8. What has that challenge cost you in the past? Time, money, energy, friends, family, career?

    _____

    _____

    _____

    _____

9. What will that challenge cost you in the future?

    _____

    _____

    _____

    _____

10. What would it be worth to you to transform that challenge right now?

_____

_____

_____

_____

Armed with all of this new knowledge you are now ready to enjoy a healthier and happier life. You have your vision and your goal and are set to complete the journey of reaching your ideal weight.

To kick start your results you need to start changing your old habits. In order to change your old habits you need to begin a daily program of forming new habits. You may find that you can't stick to this kick start plan or feel that it won't work for you. That's just because your mind doesn't like change.

Follow this plan for a minimum of 30 days and you will find that you will be on the path to success. It will take a few minutes a day to create your new habits and keep you on track. Thoughts lead to feelings, which lead to actions, which lead to results. The time is now, get started today!

Kick Start Plan™

Start each day by doing the exercises on the following pages. Make this the first thing you do every day. Do this for the next 30 days or more. You will have amazing results if you continue this for 90 days. Your new positive habits will form and you will have gained self confidence, self esteem and increased the desire to reach your goal.

Day 1

Set an intention for the day. What one thing will you do to help you on your journey to reach your ideal weight?

_____

_____

_____

_____

_____

Take 10 minutes to visualize what you will see, hear and feel when you reach your ideal weight. Write down how this makes you feel.

_____

_____

_____

_____

_____

Day 2

Set an intention for the day. What one thing will you do to help you on your journey to reach your ideal weight?

_____

_____

_____

_____

_____

State your SMART Goal out loud for 1 minute. What did you see, hear and feel while you were saying it?

_____

_____

_____

_____

_____

Day 3

Set an intention for the day. What one thing will you do to help you on your journey to reach your ideal weight?

_____

_____

_____

_____

_____

Acknowledge 3 things you are grateful for.

_____

_____

_____

_____

_____

Day 4

Set an intention for the day. What one thing will you do to help you on your journey to reach your ideal weight?

_____

_____

_____

_____

_____

List 3 reasons you deserve to reach your ideal weight.

_____

_____

_____

_____

_____

Day 5

Set an intention for the day. What one thing will you do to help you on your journey to reach your ideal weight?

_____

_____

_____

_____

_____

List 3 reasons why you want to reach your ideal weight.

_____

_____

_____

_____

_____

Day 6

Set an intention for the day. What one thing will you do to help you on your journey to reach your ideal weight?

_____

_____

_____

_____

_____

List 3 people who will benefit from you reaching your ideal weight.

_____

_____

_____

_____

_____

Day 7

Set an intention for the day. What one thing will you do to help you on your journey to reach your ideal weight?

_____

_____

_____

_____

_____

Choose one action that challenges you and that you've been avoiding. Take that action today. Write down how you felt after you accomplished it.

_____

_____

_____

_____

_____

Day 8

Set an intention for the day. What one thing will you do to help you on your journey to reach your ideal weight?

_____

_____

_____

_____

_____

Write down your goal weight. Read it out loud for 1 minute in the statement "I am _____ pounds." Write down how it makes you feel to say you are at your ideal weight.

_____

_____

_____

_____

_____

Day 9

Set an intention for the day. What one thing will you do to help you on your journey to reach your ideal weight?

_____

_____

_____

_____

_____

Write down how you will feel when you reach your ideal weight. How will you celebrate reaching your goal?

_____

_____

_____

_____

_____

Day 10

Set an intention for the day. What one thing will you do to help you on your journey to reach your ideal weight?

_____
_____
_____
_____
_____

List 3 successes you accomplished yesterday. How does that make you feel?

_____
_____
_____
_____
_____

Day 11

Set an intention for the day. What one thing will you do to help you on your journey to reach your ideal weight?

_____

_____

_____

_____

_____

Choose one person who has helped you on your weight loss goal and state 3 reasons why you appreciate them.

_____

_____

_____

_____

_____

Day 12

Set an intention for the day. What one thing will you do to help you on your journey to reach your ideal weight?

_____

_____

_____

_____

_____

Describe one obstacle you have faced reaching your ideal weight. How did you overcome it? How did that make you feel?

_____

_____

_____

_____

_____

Day 13

Set an intention for the day. What one thing will you do to help you on your journey to reach your ideal weight?

_____

_____

_____

_____

_____

Do one thing today to push you outside of your comfort zone. Describe how it makes you feel.

_____

_____

_____

_____

_____

Day 14

Set an intention for the day. What one thing will you do to help you on your journey to reach your ideal weight?

_____

_____

_____

_____

_____

Look at your results so far. Determine one thing you haven't done yet in order to get you to the next step. Do it today. Write down how accomplishing it makes you feel.

_____

_____

_____

_____

_____

Day 15

Go back to Day 1 and begin the process again for the next 14 days. Follow this action plan and you will be more successful and happier with your progress. Acknowledge your accomplishments and the hard work you put in. Share your success and enjoy the results you have achieved.

Congratulations on your new beginning!

Remember to visit:
www.moniquebartlett.com/workshops and register for the **Kick Start For Weight Loss Program**.

To get a FREE download of the Kick Start Plan go to:
www.kickstartforweightloss.com/free-tools

Recommended Resources

A percentage of the proceeds from this book will be going to:

Heart Lake Community Food Cupboard
85 Sandalwood Parkway E, Brampton, Ontario, L6Z 4S3

Heart Lake Community Food Cupboard (HLCFC) is a non-denominational food cupboard working towards providing assistance to those in need in the under serviced areas of Brampton, Ontario.

This initiative began operation October, 2012 at Heart Lake United Church in Brampton and is operated entirely by volunteers.

HLCFC's primary funder is Moore Brothers Transport – a local business dedicated to giving back to its community. Food has been donated by various corporations, schools, local churches, food drives and individuals. HLCFC currently does not receive funding from any municipal, provincial or federal government.

HLCFC is located at the Heart Lake United Church and is open *by appointment only* on Sunday (from 12:30pm -2:00pm) and Wednesday evenings (from 7:00pm-9:00pm).

Monetary and food donations are always welcome. We also need volunteers. Please call (905) 846-4519 or email **hlcfc@live.com** for more information on how you can be involved.

The
Millionaire Mind
Intensive

T. Harv Eker is author of the #1 NY Times bestselling book, Secrets of the Millionaire Mind, and his programs have really helped me, as well as hundreds of thousands of people all over the world. You can learn to **RESET** your blueprint for a higher level of success.

There are events scheduled in cities all across the US and Canada. They're even offering **Free General Seating** registration!

Go to
http://kickstartforweightloss.com/MillionaireMind
and register today!

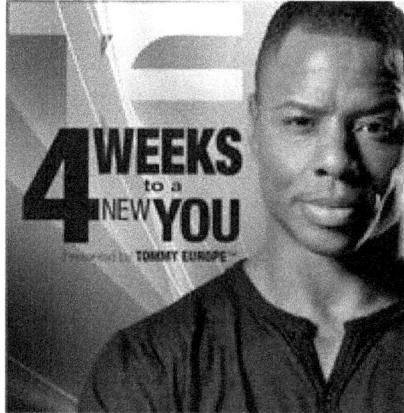

Tommy Europe Fitness (TEF) is an International fitness company that is run by one of Canada's most in-demand fitness experts, Tommy Europe™.

Tommy is best known as the tough love personal trainer, and television host of the "The Last 10 Pounds Bootcamp", and "Bulging Brides."

If your goal is to **upgrade your fitness with a proven plan**, Tommy helps women just like you, bust through plateaus, improve your overall Health & Fitness levels, get more toned, and permanently lose inches & pounds.

Regardless of your current health and fitness level, Tommy will give you all of the tools, expertise, and the right **PLAN** to make your total body transformation a **SUCCESS**!

Go to **http://kickstartforweightloss.com/TommyEurope**
and register today!

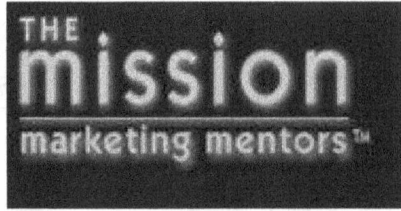

Are you a professional, expert, author or speaker who has a mission, calling or positive purpose you are accomplishing through your practice or business?

Take the **Free Ultimate Client Magnet** mini course that will teach you the steps to create a book that attracts new clients and generates multiple income streams in as few as 90 days.

Go to
http://kickstartforweightloss.com/missionmarketing
and register today!

Know you are
MEANT for MORE?
Not sure how to get there?
Check this out!

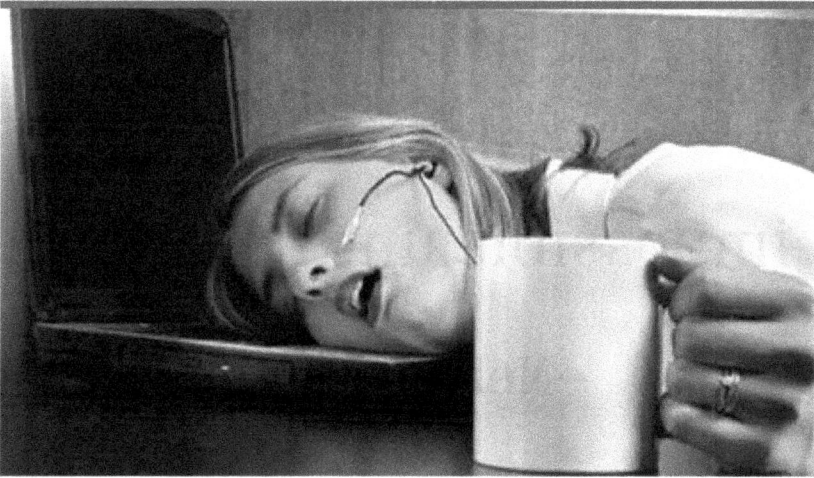

Sometimes when you are struggling with one area of your life it transcends into other areas. Catch Fire University is a program for which I have personally read this book & taken the Online Course! Two words: **LIFE CHANGING!** Take advantage, you can get **BOTH 4 FREE** right now!

Go to **http://kickstartforweightloss.com/catchfire**
and register for the online course today!

"It always seems impossible until it's done."

~Nelson Mandela

Listen to the <u>Kick Start For Weight Loss</u> Podcast On iTunes

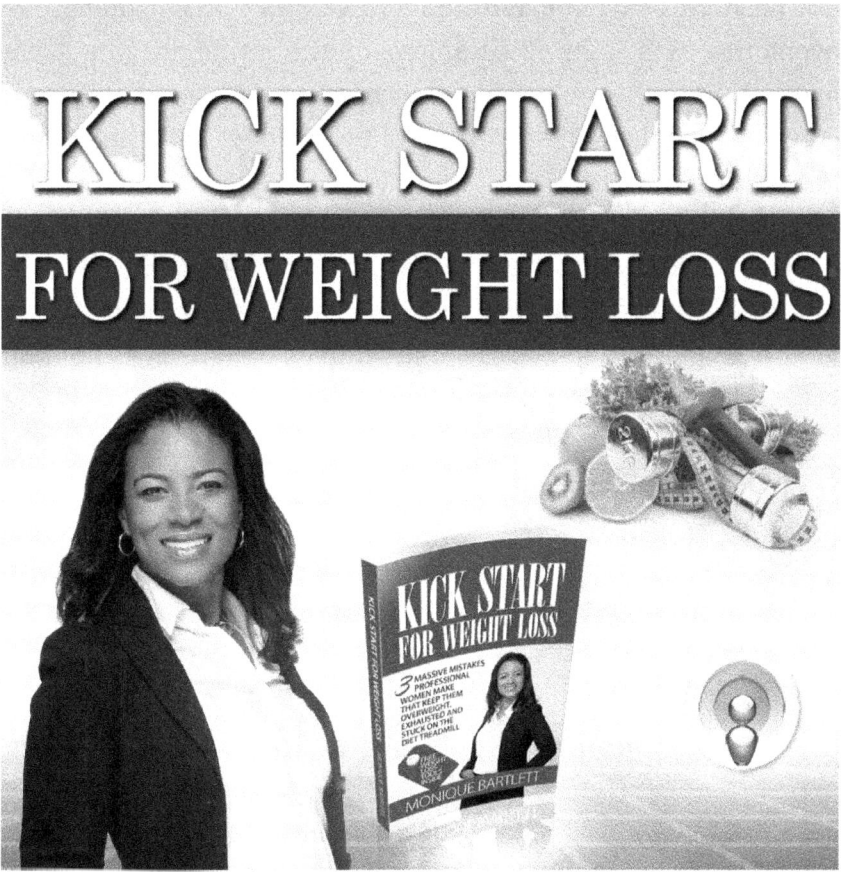

Kick Start for Women Workshop™

Create the Mindset for Positive Results

The **Kick Start for Women Workshop™** is an interactive event that will help you implement the strategies you have learned in this book. The environment is stimulating and supportive and will help you make the changes you need to get the results you want.

You will be given practical tools to anchor the things you have learned, even after the workshop is over. If you are looking for a breakthrough in your life and are looking to set your boundaries and release yourself from whatever is holding you back, this workshop is for you.

This workshop will open your eyes and your mind to make your ideal weight a reality.

For more information call:
1-647-955-5646 or 1-866-680-1266

You can also send an email to:
monique@moniquebartlett.com

Visit my website at:
www.moniquebartlett.com/workshops

Want More Income?

Monique Bartlett regularly partners with individuals to create multiple sources of income. Several opportunities are available such as joint ventures, partnerships, speaking and training. If you are serious about achieving a higher income and more time freedom, then contact Monique today.

Call **1-647-955-5646 or 1-866-680-1266**

You can also send an email to:
monique@moniquebartlett.com

Sources Consulted

Schoenfeld, Brad. *Sculpting Her Body Perfect,* Third Edition Human Kinetics MMVIII

Redman, Kim. *Designing Your Destiny™ Training Manual* Creatrix Transformational Solutions Inc. Ver. 6.0 MMXII

Kennedy, Lori. WOW Professional Certification Manual PLNW Inc. 2013 and Beyond MMXIIII

Health Canada. www.healthcanada.gc.ca/eatwell-beactive Accessed January MMXIII

Galam. *Yoga Now Nutrition Plan MMV*

Tooley Transformation Training MMXIII

Krasner, Dr. A.M. *The Wizard Within,* Third Edition American Board of Hypnotherapy Press MMI

"It's not about being the best; it's about doing your best."

~Arlene Dickinson

"Nothing will work unless you do."

~Maya Angelou

About The Author

Monique Bartlett is an author, speaker and coach.

Her story is compelling as she went from overweight to fit by using her can do attitude. Every woman who is overweight, exhausted and stuck on the diet treadmill can relate to Monique because if she can do it, you can do it too!

Her style is professional and engaging bringing with it laughter and lightheartedness. Monique is also a regular columnist and contributor to various newspapers.

Her ideas are practical strategies that will make you believe in yourself and show you that you knew how to do it all along. You just needed some help to realize it.

Monique can be reached in Toronto, Ontario, Canada at **1-647-955-5646** or **1-866-680-1266.**

You can also send an email to: **monique@moniquebartlett.com** or find her on Social Media at:

Facebook: www.facebook.com/MoniqueBartlettAuthor
Twitter: @MoniqueBart
LinkdedIn: Monique Bartlett
Pinterest: Monique Bartlett
You Tube: Monique Bartlett

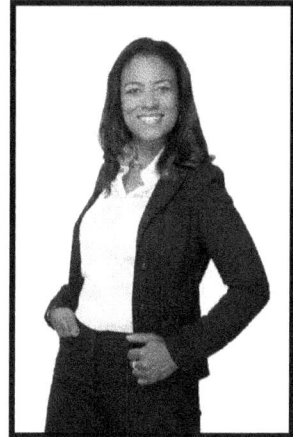

For more information on how to participate in one of Monique's workshops or to hire her as a speaker, visit her website at: **www.moniquebartlett.com**

Notes

Notes

Notes

Notes

www.ingramcontent.com/pod-product-compliance
Lightning Source LLC
Chambersburg PA
CBHW050543280326
41933CB00011B/1701